I0414260

NCD
Beef Stroganoff

40% carbs 30% fat 30% protein and 500 calories

Number Crunch Diet Publications

ABC Water and the Number Crunch Diet
12 Changes A Year – Reality-Show Recipes

12 Changes A Year – Volume 3
the recipe book to the Number Crunch Diet
You have to crunch the numbers to see what you're really eating.

Reality-Show RECIPES
12 Changes A Year – Vol. 1, 2, & 3
for the person who likes it real

Vision Is Possible
Improve your vision and get a facelift for free!
an original vision program targeting your Eye Lids

RAW MILK
the legal "Anabolic Steroid" for
common-sense Californians

GOOD Bacteria – Your Other Bodypart
looking deeper into your body's 2nd brain

NCD Lactose Intolerance Protocol
the Number Crunch Diet method to wean
yourself back on to milk

September 23, 2015 – The Rapture
Even if this date is wrong, you'll be ready for the next one.
What group are you in?

NCD Orange Shake
mmm! mmm! mmm!
The Number Crunch Diet uses real foods for flavor.

CONTENTS

To scroll through all 50 recipes, please visit

http://www.CreateSpace.com/6415388

Edits & Format

You will notice oddities in punctuation, spelling, syntax, and perhaps even semantics, within this book. Feel free to let me know, but some of it is done for brevity or to shift emphasis. I use capitals where I see fit, to grab your attention and make it stand out, and I also remove capitals when I don't think they are deserving of them, or to remove emphasis after first usage, i.e., Pyrex becomes pyrex. And french bread, brussels sprouts, and english cucumbers, are spelled lowercase, as we are not going to "link" a European vacation to our food and eating.

Secondly, I will unhyphenate to create rhythm. Grammatically, two or more words that function as an adjective before a noun are supposed to be hyphenated. That's fine. A million-dollar smile, is the adjective "million-dollar" describing the smile. However, this can get redundant after a while, 1&2 3, 1&2 3, 1&2 3. The noun gets all the attention. But what if you want the adjectives to have the emphasis? After all, the adjectives are the descriptive words. So, I will drop the hyphens to allow the adjectives equal emphasis, and to change the pace of the sentence a bit. So if there are no hyphens, read it slower and evenly, one two three four five six seven. A "step-by-step solution" sounds a bit skippy and simplistic, whereas, a "step by step solution" is said slower and sounds more methodical. Hyphenating two words, or joining two words as a compound word, reduces their individual meanings.

With regard to fastfood, healthfood, and seasalt, it's time for these words to evolve into compound words, so the trend starts here.

There are also some fragmented sentences, subject-verb disagreements, and singular/plural violations. When "correcting" certain of these sentences, they lost their emphasis and punch, so I kept them as is.

In the past I've been guilty of judging other author's sentences, only to reread it with the commas, pauses, and then it made perfect sense. So, if there's a comma, then pause, as you may not get to pause later in the sentence. If there's no comma, then don't pause and read it all as one.

I pose questions, but without question marks. Some are rhetorical, but some are to make you Ponder. Great word. Ponder. If you see a question mark at the end, then it requires an answer. If there's no question mark, then you can just say, yeah, no, or hm.

As I read comments made on the internet, I have come to the acceptance that an incomplete sentence or a prepositional phrase can actually stand alone as a sentence. For example, the comment, "Yes. In so many ways." A period instead of a comma, allows for a longer pause between the two, and so this is more accurately how someone might speak it. So a period can be used as a long pause, instead of "Yes, in so many ways."

The spelling of HomeGoods, PubMed, and others, has become common. You can now join two words and keep the capital.

Written English continues to change, people using it, customize the language to reflect exactly how they would speak it. It's a bit like ballroom dancing, the person leading gets to decide the movements and the pace, and each partner you dance with will use different movements and different paces. That said, I hope you enjoy this dance…

God Bless.

Steven Barry

You have to crunch the numbers to see what you're really eating.

Begin today and forever be in control of the numbers you're eating.

When you take control of the numbers, you take control of your weight.

Number Crunch Diet Publications – always profanity free

CHAPTER 1

Introduction

Woohoo!

Welcome to the Number Crunch Diet – Complete Nutrition, Maximum Freedom, Total Control. It's really the "All Your Dreams Come True Control Freak" diet. With a side of entertainment! But seriously, if you've tried the no-meat diet, or the no-carb diet, or the no-this diet no-that diet, then you are in for a treat. The NCD says: Eat it, and get it out of your system. And only the NCD says this.

In fact, after you've eaten everything you want, over and over again, you come to the place where – You Don't Want Anything Anymore. And you simply eat to supply your body with nutrition and energy. Of course there are some "rules", principles, and a brief summary will be provided in the next chapter.

Whereas the main book, *ABC Water and the Number Crunch Diet*, and the three cookbooks, *12 Changes A Year, Volumes 1, 2, and 3*, read like one giant 1000-page book, (so you can't really jump in anywhere and expect to fully understand it all, as it builds and flows from chapter to chapter), conversely, these NCD booklets are stand alone, you can read any one of the 50 booklets in any order.

Are you ready! I know you are! Let's pump this sucker out and get to it, but first we need "The Basics".

Chapter 2

The Basics

On the NCD, we count calories by counting pre-counted meals. Meaning that, you make a recipe, divide it up, and each serving, or meal, is 500 calories. The word "snack" means 250 calories.

Meal = 500
Snack = 250

You will only eat NCD meals and NCD snacks. So if you have 4 meals a day, you've had 4x500=2000 calories a day. If you have 5 meals a day, you've had 5x500=2500 calories a day. Six meals a day, 3000 calories. Seven meals, 3500 calories, and so on. For those of you that work physical jobs, you work on a fishing boat, or an oil rig, or you do yardwork 8-10 hours a day, then 4000 and 5000 and even 6000 calories a day is likely what your intake needs are. For these people, we have D-Meals, Double Meals, a double meal for breakfast, a meal and a shake for lunch, a double meal late-afternoon, and a double meal in the evening, 4x1000=4000.

If you're a woman working an office job, then your day might look like this:
Breakfast – 500
break – 250
Lunch – 500
break – 250
Dinner – 500

2000 calories a day, spread out throughout the day, 2-3-4 hours apart. There are lots of options for how you can consume your daily calories, and how to cut calories, and for that you will have to read the main books. But that gives you, The Basics.

Next, we will take a close look at the label of every food product we purchase, as that food is going into your body, and your body has to make new cells from that food, or detoxify any of the bad stuff that's in it. Preachers will say, the Bible is the "good news", but when it comes to your body, the "good news" is your liver. On the NCD we are allowed bad ingredients Rarely to Occasionally only. Not in moderation. The NCD says, "Moderation is too much." And, if you're a wine drinker, you need to cut that out. Drinking alcohol is a scam. It dehydrates your body and makes you age. Pomegranate juice contains just as much polyphenols and resveratrol as wine, as does simple grape juice. The NCD has a no alcohol rule. See the NCD Chicken Alfredo recipe for how to wean yourself off of red wine.

Young people, you are being scammed by the media and our culture into thinking that drinking alcohol and partying is fun. It's not. Do it, try it, and then move on. They are fooling you. You lose. The NCD is a health diet, so expect some lecturing. You will never fulfill your potential and purpose for being born if you waste your time drinking and partying on your days off. So, get busy. Set some goals. And focus in on them, like a laser beam. :)

Of all the people out there that read books, I would say 80% are women, so men, you've got some catching up to do.

And by books, I mean useful material, self-help, self-improvement. Christians spend time reading the Bible, and then call into a radio program crying because they've been diagnosed with cancer and are devastated and helpless. When someone says, "pray for me," hand them a self-help book and tell them to read their way out of their situation and trial. God has never failed me, He has always taken me through, BUT, I had to take action, I had to do it. He guides, you do.

Reading results in knowledge, then from there you can take Action.

Faith is not: God will come through. Faith is: God will guide your footsteps, and if you do it, you will come through. But in order to take action, you first need ample knowledge about your situation, otherwise, you are "destroyed", Hosea 4:6.

The NCD is a holistic diet, body mind soul spirit, whole body.

Although most of the recipes are 40 30 30, the NCD utilizes other macro percents as well, this is outlined in the main books. However, your day-in day-out macros should be 40 30 30. Everything you put in your mouth will be 40 30 30. Later, if you want to use different macros for different situation, then absolutely, go-for-it. But to start, just stick to 40 30 30. It's steady and stable, almost a-third a-third a-third, with a slight tip towards the carbs. If you want to argue or debate me on macro percents, read the main books first. I'm giving you the basics here.

So again, no bag of chips as a snack, everything you put in your mouth will be 40 30 30, and either 500 calories, or half, 250.

There aren't a lot of snack recipes on the NCD, so when you want a snack, just have half a meal. The NCD soups are great for cutting calories. They are 250 calories, but they fill you up like a 500 calorie meal. So, have the NCD French Onion soup for breakfast, and cut your breakfast calories from 500 to 250. But regular soups won't do it, as they are not 40 30 30.

The macro ratios are the key.

Once you begin to eat only pre-counted meals and snacks, then you can easily track your daily calories, as previously discussed. And once you know your calorie requirement, then you have control.

To do this, you must make a goal that you will continue to build your recipe repertoire until 100% of your eating comes from homemade meals you prepare yourself. No meals of unknown calories. This needs to be your goal. In the beginning, if you are in a pinch, you can, for example, walk over to the vending machine at work and have a regular-sized snickers bar, about 280 calories, just say 250. So this is your midmorning snack. But your goal is to prepare meals, all 40 30 30 and 500, and then bring meals and half-meals (snacks) to work so that 100% of your eating is 40 30 30.

Again, the reasons and the options are explained in the main books.

Trust me, I've been working on this diet for 15 years, perfecting the principles, expanding the options, and weeding out bad for good.

The Number Crunch Diet is not a get-thin-quick scheme. The recipe books are titled 12 Changes A Year on purpose, so, once a month, start a new recipe, make it again, then, next month repeat the cycle. At the end of one year, you should have 12 recipes in your repertoire. At the end of two years, 24 recipes, and at the end of three years, 36 recipes. Bingo! You're there. Goal: achieved. You will be eating 100% of your food from homemade meals you prepare yourself, from well-chosen grocery store items.

Hence, Complete Nutrition – Maximum Freedom – Total Control.

There's more that needs to be said, but let's just jump in and start, you will figure out the rest as you go. The best way to learn is to just, jump in. Dog paddle until you can swim! Let's go!

Chapter 3

The Items

The items you select to eat are important, as is how you cook them. You are what you eat, was true yesterday, is true today, and will still be true tomorrow.

If you eat animal muscle (meat), with the preservative sodium nitrite, you end up with nitrosamides (cancer).

If you cook that animal muscle (meat) at high temperatures and char it, burn it, until it's got black marks, you create polycyclic aromatic hydrocarbons (plastics).

Throw in a side of french fries deep fried in oil at 425°F, and you're eating acrylamides (cancer).

And if you chase that charred burger patty or flame-broiled chicken with a diet soft drink (aspartame), you create heterocyclic amines.

So the NCD takes a close look at what we are eating, we read the entire label:
1. the ingredients list
2. the nutrition facts numbers
3. the label bragging ("our product is …")

The fastest way to cut out all of those cancer-causing compounds listed above, is to eat your food RAW, the NCD is about 80% raw.

This recipe requires about 8 different items, and it makes 16 meals.
1. egg noodles
2. beef x4
3. onion
4. mushrooms x4
5. beef broth, butter, flour (the gravy)
6. sour cream (regular & lite)
7. NCD breadsticks
8. parsley

As stated in the main books, if you live in California, well lucky you, as you will recognize these supermarkets, but clearly, I cannot shop for items in every city in the world and tell you where to go. You will have to search for the same or similar items in your area.

1. American Beauty Wide Egg Noodles, Food Maxx market, 32oz 2lb 907g, buy 1 bag, $2.79 on sale ($3.79 regular price).
Ingredients: durum flour (wheat), dried egg yolks or eggs, niacin, ferrous sulfate (iron), thiamine mononitrate, riboflavin, folic acid.

So we see it's refined. They've refined out the iron and B vitamins, and then added them back in. Otherwise, fine. No natural flavors, that's important. These noodles are "fun carbs".

The nutrition facts for this item (in the United States) looks like this:

2oz 56 grams
Servings per container, about 16
Calories per serving = 210
Calories of Fat = 25
Fat = 2.5g
Saturated Fat = 0.5g
Trans Fat = 0g
Cholesterol = 65mg (milligrams)
Sodium = 5mg
Carbohydrate = 38g
Fiber = 2g

Sugar = 2g
Protein = 8g

People in Canada, Australia, the UK and elsewhere, your label may or may not have all these listed, or it may say Kcal, Kilo calories. Don't worry, just follow along. I like the U.S. nutrition facts label the best, however, they are planning on changing it and the proposed new label is…not that great.

So as you can see, the label has two units of measure, calories and grams. On the NCD we convert grams into calories, see below:

Fat grams to calories = times by 9
Carb grams to calories = times by 4
Protein grams to calories = times by 4

So, 9 4 4.

Also, the nutrition facts list the fat, then the carbs, then the protein. However, when we refer to the macro percents, the order is carbs fat protein.

40 30 30 is Carbs Fat Protein, so just be aware that the label has the Fat first.

None of the NCD recipes contain trans fat, so you won't see that number again. And saturated fat and cholesterol are both within normal limits on the NCD, so you won't see those again either.

So, I'm going to recrunch the label into calories, and write it all on one line. E=210 F=25 Na=5 CHO=152 f=8 s=8 Prot=32 T=209.

E = Energy, in calories
F = Fat, in calories
Na = sodium, in milligrams
CHO = Carbs, in calories
f = fiber, in calories
s = sugar, in calories

Prot = Protein, in calories
T = the total calories (Fat + Carbs + Protein)
T-f = T (total calories, fat+carbs+prot) minus the fiber

I go over this in full detail in the main books, but for this recipe, you don't really need to master all the calculations and numbers, but you should try to familiarize yourself with them. It's just one of the things in life a person should know and be familiar with.

Before we move on, I want you to notice that the calories are given at the top (210), but you can calculate it yourself by adding together the three items that have calories, Fat Carbs Protein (209).

This is how we double-check the accuracy of the label, E and T should match, or be close.

T-f. T is the total calories (fat+carbs+prot), and f is the fiber calories. Fiber comes in two forms, soluble and insoluble. The insoluble fiber doesn't enter your body, it stays within the colon, thereby, adding bulk to your stool. The soluble fiber gets absorbed into your body, but it creates a gel gelatin-like matrix that slows down the release of sugar into the bloodstream.

On the NCD, we subtract the fiber calories from our numbers.

So T-f is total calories minus the fiber, in this case, 209-8=201.

We also subtract the fiber from the carbs number, in this case, 152-8=144, and we call this number nCHO, net carbohydrates.

Lastly, we look at the macro percents of each food item. 40 30 30 is the macro percent of the meal, but each food item has its own percents.

To calculate the percent of something, you take the portion and divide it by the whole, times 100. With this food item, we have 25/209x100=12% fat, 152/209x100=73% carbs, and 32/209x100 =15% protein, 73 12 15.

3   Items

We have 3 things that make up the whole. Fats Carbs Protein

And they add up to the total calories, E, Energy. (and T)

I'll stop there, as I don't want to go too deep. It is all covered in progressive steps, with repetition, so that you will be a number crunch expert at the end. Your kids will be amazed by you!

And again, I've simplified the statements and rounded off the numbers. This is a booklet, not a book.

Now let's look at the third and final part of our food item, the label bragging. If you shop at the healthfood store, you will immediately notice that the food items have a lot of label bragging, and often true and important scientific facts. Many companies are catching on that in order to be competitive, they have to brag about their product and tell you what's good in it and why you should buy theirs over other brands. Some bragging is fake, for example, ketchup or Worcestershire sauce saying "fat free" on the label. Everyone knows that. Plus good fats are good for you, so a diet that is "fat free" is not a healthy diet. And we all know this now.

Fat Free is one of the many mainstream media scams. In the 1990s, doctors put their overweight patients on fat-free diets, which can only mean one thing – you eat more carbs. One woman I worked with said when she went back to her doctor a month later, she had gained 5 pounds.

Fat Free also means dry skin, as your cell membranes are dry.

Saturated fat is actually a great fat for soft hair and soft skin.™

And saturated fat is a natural fat, it's unprocessed. All vegetable oils, including olive oil, are processed.

On the NCD we eat 30% fat, and a balance of plant & animal fats.

Keep in mind that you cannot make two kinds of fat; omega-3 flax, and fish fat DHA EPA. I encourage you to read up on this fully.

Our egg noodles are not really nutritious, just refined pasta. But we will get nutrition in the beef, onion, mushrooms, etc.

One-sixteenth of 32oz is 2oz, so our numbers are the same as the nutrition facts on page 7 and 8.

Be sure to buy WIDE egg noodles. They are available at most stores. And don't use three 12oz bags, as that's 36 ounces.

2. Ground Beef 96/4 Extra Lean, Trader Joe's, 16oz 454g, buy 4 x $5.49 = $21.96. This 96/4 extra lean ground beef is available at most stores, and Smart & Final has a 2-pound size for $10.99.

The NCD only uses 96% lean 4% fat ground beef, never 90/10 or 85/15 or 80/20, and you will see why, next.

4oz 113g
Servings per container 4
E=130cal
F=40cal
total Fat = 4g (x9 = 36cal) (close to 40)
SF=2g (x9=18calories of saturated fat, not a problem)
Chol=60mg (animal foods are where we get cholesterol from)
Na=65mg
CHO=0
f=0
s=0
Prot=21g (x4=84cal)
T=40+0+84=124cal (close to E=130 above)

Notice that the fat is given in calories (40), and in grams (4g). On the NCD, we use the Fat Cals number (40cal), and not the grams number, (4gx9cal=36cal).

And then our percents are, 40/124x100=32% fat, 0% carbs, 84/124x100=68% protein, 0 32 68.

Extra Lean ground beef is about 70 30 protein and fat.

So even though the label says 4% fat, we can see that it is really 32% fat by calories, about one-third fat.

NCD Beef-Labeling Exposed™
96% lean 4% fat = 32% fat by calories, energy
90% lean 10% fat (E=200 F=100) = 50% fat by calories
85% lean 15% fat (E=240 F=150) = 62.5% fat
80% lean 20% fat is 69% fat (E=290 F=200, 200/290x100=69%)
Some of the 80/20 beef packs "brag" about being 20% fat, liars.

Well, they will say, "We aren't lying, we are allowed to state it like this because of the way the regulations are written."

You will encounter this everywhere in life. Things are allowed to be written deceptively, but the truth is quite different than what they say.

We are having 4oz per meal, so exactly as stated on the nutrition facts above.

3. Organic Beef Broth, Trader Joe's, 32 fl oz 946mL carton, $2.49. Ingredients: organic beef stock (water, organic beef), sea salt, organic beef stock flavor (organic beef stock, water, organic honey, organic tomato paste, organic onion puree, flavor, organic dextrose, organic molasses, organic soybean oil), organic evaporated cane sugar, organic garlic powder, organic onion powder, organic caramel color.

That's a lot of organic, good. They even disclose what is in the beef stock flavor, nice. Even the caramel color is organic. There is one word, "flavor", in the beef stock flavor that is not organic, but overall, a good product. Dextrose is glucose.

The nutrition facts say:
1 cup (8oz 240mL)
Servings per container 4

E=15cal
F=0cal
Na=570mg
CHO=1g (x4=4cal)
f=0
s<1g (zero) (the "<" sign looks like an L, for Less than)
Prot=2g (x4=8cal)
T=0+4+8=12cal
33 0 67 (33% carbs, 0% fat, 67% protein)

The label brags that it is made from the finest beef stock and with top quality ingredients, and we can see that this is true.

We will have 2oz per meal, so we have to recrunch the nutrition facts, 2oz/8oz=0.25, so we multiply the label by 0.25, E=4 F=0 Na=140 CHO=1 Prot=2 T=3.

4.   Fresh Mushrooms, Food Maxx, 16oz 454g, buy 4, $2.99x4=$11.96. We will have 4oz per meal, so the cost is 75 cents per meal, just for the mushrooms. Mushrooms have doubled in price. That means, they must be good for you.

Be sure to pick full and heavy packages, and dig to the back of the shelf for the freshest available.

We are going to slice them, but I don't recommend buying sliced mushrooms as they have been sliced 1-2 days ago. Just buy whole mushrooms and slice them yourself so they are fresh looking.

On the NCD, we don't count the vegetables as they are "free", but let's look at the numbers just so you know.

3oz 85g
E=20
F=0
Na=15
K=300 (300 milligrams of potassium per 3oz serving, nice)
CHO=3gx4=12cal

f=1gx4=4cal
s=0
Prot=3gx4=12cal
T=24
50% carbs and 50% protein

The label also says 100% of the RDA for vitamin D. That means that 3oz of mushrooms have 400 IUs of vitamin D. Amazing. The label also goes on to say that they are a good source of B vitamins, the antioxidant selenium (a mineral), and 15% the RDA of copper.

So now we know why they cost so much. Nutrition.

The other brand of mushrooms I bought says 4% the RDA for vitamin D, and you will see inconsistencies on labels, but just start reading them. (RDA, Recommended Daily Allowance)

Since we are having 4oz, then E=27 K=400 CHO=16 Prot=16.

5. Yellow Onion, "Spanish" Onion, we want 16oz of onion, so buy 1.2 lbs (almost one-and-a-quarter pounds), and so when we cut off the ends and remove one layer of peel, we'll have 16oz of onion.

At Food Maxx, they are 47 cents /lb, so 56 cents total.

6a. Sour Cream, 16oz 454g, Daisy brand, Food Maxx, $2.39. Ingredients: grade A cultured cream. One ingredient. Trader Joe's is $1.69, but it lists several ingredients. 2T 30g E=60 F=45

6b. Lite Sour Cream, 16oz 454g, Daisy brand, Food Maxx, $2.39. Ingredients: cream, skim milk, vitamin A. Again, TJs brand is cheaper, but it has modified food starch, guar gum, carrageenan, sodium phosphate, sodium citrate, locust bean gum, etc.

2T (tablespoons) 30g E=40 F=25 (so it's lite, less calories and fat).

We will mix these two containers of sour cream together and divide by 16, E=95 F=66 SF=47 Chol=28 Na=38 CHO=11 Pro=11.

7.   King Arthur Flour, 100% hard red whole wheat flour, 5lb 2.27Kg bag, S&F $4.79, or FM, Never Bleached, Never Bromated, Non-GMO (not genetically modified).

The NF says $1/4^{th}$ cup 30g E=100 F=5 CHO=20g f=4g s=0 Pro=4g, and we will use 60g for the batch of 16 meals, so one meal is E=13 F=1 CHO=10 f=2 Prot=2.

On the NCD, a whole grain has to have a double-digit fiber percent. Let's crunch it. The fiber is 4g so 16 calories, and T=101 (5+80+16), so 16÷101x100=15.8% or 16%. Double digit percent fiber, so it's a true whole grain.

Notice that the egg noodles are 4% fiber, a refined grain, 2gx4=8, and T=209, so 8÷209x100=3.8%=4%.

8.   Sprouted Flourless Whole Wheat Berry Bread, Trader Joe's, 24oz 680g, $3.49. Ingredients: sprouted organic whole wheat berries, filtered water, wheat gluten, organic dates, fresh yeast, sea salt, organic raisins, soy lecithin (emulsifier), cultured wheat.

1 slice 34g E=80 F=0 Na=160 CHO=15gx4=60 f=2g s=2g Pro=5g.

What's the percent fiber?

2gx4=8 ÷ 80 = 0.1 x100 = 10% fiber, double digit.

The label used to mention glycemic index and glycemic load, (two very important factors used on the NCD). 40 30 30 is a measured glycemic load.

We will have 2/3rds of a slice per meal, E=57 F=0 Na=107 CHO=40 f=5 s=5 Prot=13 T=53.

NCD Breadsticks™
The loaf is 20 slices, so remove them from the bag and place them in two stacks of 10, face down on the counter. So the two end pieces are facing you. Take your breadknife, and saw through the

stack of 10, about 1¼ inches from the edge, and repeat, sawing through the stack about 1¼ inches from the edge. You will now have 30 strips of bread, 30 "breadsticks". Repeat with the other stack.

You will have 2 breadsticks per meal, so 16 meals is 32 breadsticks, with 28 breadsticks left over. Use them to make NCD French Onion Soup.

To make the breadsticks hard, place them in a container in the fridge. I use two ice-cube white plastic containers, and just place them in the containers with some space between them and they will dry out and harden as the days go by. They will be completely hard (like breadsticks) in two weeks, so if you want hard crunchy breadsticks, then make them two weeks in advance.

See the rear cover of the NCD Beef & Rice recipe booklet for how these breadsticks appear in my refrigerator.

9. Organic Butter, Trader Joe's, 16oz 454g, unsalted, $4.99.
Ingredients: pasteurized organic sweet cream (milk), lactic acid.

1T 14g E=100 SF=7gx9=63cal Chol=30 Na=0 CHO=0 Prot=0.

We will use 38g for the batch of 16 meals, so each meal will be E=17 F=17 SF=11 Chol=5. Butter is an animal fat, and 63% saturated fat, 63/100x100. But there is nothing bad about saturated fat, as long as you are also getting plant fats.

And especially fish fat (cod liver oil), and flax seeds (omega-3).

10.   And lastly, parsley, one fresh organic bunch, Cal-Organic brand, Albertsons supermarket, 99 cents. I have also purchased the nonorganic parsley at Food Maxx and it was fine, no pesticide suds when I washed it, and no stomach gurgling from fungicides.

Okay, let's hit the kitchen and put this all together.

Chapter 4

Assembly

The noodles are the tricky part as they will glue together if you don't do it right, so we will make them last, then add them to the bowl of beef-onions-mushrooms, so that they don't stick together.

Place a large skillet on the counter and grab your mushroom slicer, Ontel brand, The Mushroom Xpress, as seen on TV. Transfer all four packs of mushrooms to a large bowl, place 2-3 mushrooms in your hand and rinse them, flick off the water, and place them in a colander to drip.

I used to add all the mushrooms to a big bowl of hot water and wash them, flick off the water, and let drip, but they can get a bit soft if you let them stay in the water. If they are soft, they won't push through the slicer as easily. You want firm mushrooms.

Now move the colander of washed mushrooms over to the counter next to the skillet, and slice the mushrooms one by one into the skillet. Or you can use a food processor, but this mushroom slicer is actually quite fast and easy to use.

Hold the handle with your right, and angle it 45 degrees, with the right side lower and the left side higher. Now place a mushroom inside the slicer upside down, i.e., head first. Then close the top with your left hand (left thumb). Boom. It goes through. Repeat repeat repeat until you have sliced all the mushrooms.

If the mushroom doesn't go through all the way, don't worry, as the next mushroom will push it through. Just be sure your mushrooms are fresh and firm, and don't use this slicer for cheese or meats as it will dull the blades. The blades are super sharp, so this is why it's so easy, just boom boom boom boom and you're done.

You now have a skillet full of sliced mushrooms. Cover with the lid and turn it to 250°F 121°C, set a timer. At 10:00, remove the cover and mix and flip the mushrooms, then put the lid back on. At 13:00, unplug the skillet and dump the mushrooms into a colander in the sink. Let it drip a few minutes.

Now add the mushrooms to a large bowl, the NCD #5 bowl.

You don't need water to cook the mushrooms as they are 34% water, (about 1/3rd water).

DO NOT overcook the mushrooms. Set a timer and follow it.

Wash and dry the skillet, plug it in, and turn it to 250° again. Hit the timer. Add the 4 packs of ground beef, and use a plastic turner spatula to break the beef apart and mix and flip it. Keep the lid off the skillet and don't stop mixing and flipping the ground beef (and breaking it up into bits and pieces). This is your protein, so treat it with care.

At 8:00 minutes on your timer, unplug the skillet, as the ground beef will be medium-well cooked, just a slight pink remaining.

Continue to mix and flip the ground beef off heat, now pat it down and make a flat layer of cooked ground beef. At 12:00 on your timer, use your spatula to transfer the beef to the bowl with the mushrooms, holding the end of the skillet up so that the juice is at one end and stays in the skillet.

Cut the ends off the onions and remove one layer. Also, cut a cone-shaped piece out of the top of the onion where the stem was. Weigh your onions, you should have 16oz 454 grams, not more.

Using a V-slicer, slice the onion into the skillet, thick side slices. The skillet has about one cup of beef juice, so this will be enough liquid to cook the onions, (you need 1/2c of liquid to cook them).

Now carefully cut the onions into quarters, cutting in half, then the halves in half, (instead of full circles of onion slices). It doesn't have to be perfect, just cut them up without touching the skillet.

Cover with the lid, hit the timer, and set it to 250°F. Stir and mix it every 2 minutes. At 9:00, unplug the skillet, and dump this into the #5 bowl with the mushrooms and beef. Mix it some.

The Gravy
Add 38g of butter to the skillet, add the quart of beef broth, cover with the lid and turn it to high (425°F 218°C), hit the timer.

Tip. I have a bowl on my scale, so, I place my skillet on the bowl, balancing it, then turn on the scale, it reads zero, now I add butter until it says 38 grams.

At 9:00 on your timer, the broth will be rolling boiling, unplug the skillet. Now, place your wave blender pitcher in the sink, and carefully pour this broth liquid into the blender pitcher.

Tip. Be sure the pitcher bottom is screwed on tight and the rubber washer is centered on the bottom base of the pitcher.

Now place the pitcher with the hot broth on the scale and turn it on, it will read zero. Now hold a squeeze-handle sifter over the pitcher and add flour, squeezing the handle to sift the flour into the pitcher. Add another spoonful of flour to the sifter and keep sifting until it says 60 grams on your scale. Okay, now place the lid on the pitcher, securely on, place the pitcher on the blender base, and just pulse it on low for 3 seconds (a quick count to 5, 1 2 3 4 5). That's it. It's smooth. Pour this into the #5 bowl and mix it around with the mushrooms-beef-onions.

If you don't feel confident handling hot liquids, then you could add the broth to the blender cold, add the flour, then boil it. It's only 60 grams of flour so it shouldn't clump together. But on the other hand, it is about half-a-cup of flour, so I don't chance it.

The typical way is to add the flour to the hot broth in the skillet and stir, then add a bit more flour, and stir. This is too time-consuming and it is not as effective as blending in a wave blender. Just go slow and be careful when pouring hot liquids. And be sure your blender top and bottom are on tight, hold the top, and pulse on low, one, two, three. Perfect.

Okay, time to boil the egg noodles.

Clean the skillet and add one gallon of pH 5 water. This is "hard" water, pH acidic. If you are using water that has a lot of sodium and potassium minerals (soft water), then you may want to cut back on the boiling time. If you overcook the noodles, they will melt into a starchy liquid. They are delicate noodles.

My gallon of water is about 3885 grams, 4000 grams is too much water. Turn the skillet to high, 425°F, cover with the lid, and hit the timer. At 29:00 the water is boiling, so add the bag of noodles and pat them down flat with a wooden spatula so that the water is just covering them all. Cover and hit the timer.

At 4:30, the water is spurting, so open the air vent on the lid.

At 6:00, unplug the skillet, remove the cover, and dump the noodles with water into a large colander in the sink. Let it cool and drip for one minute only, not longer. If you let it sit and cool off, the noodles will glue together.

After one minute in the colander, dump the noodles into the #5 bowl and mix them with the mushrooms-beef-onions-gravy.

Now open the lite and regular sour cream containers, and add them on top of the beef stroganoff, and mix the two sour creams together, then mix the sour cream into the beef stroganoff.

If you are a NCD follower, then you have the weight of your bowls posted on your refrigerator door. My big #5 bowl is 762 grams.

Now you will want to weigh this batch of beef stroganoff, but it is almost 18 pounds, so if you have a 10-pound scale, then you have to divide it into two bowls to weigh it. I have a 10-kilogram 22-pound scale, so I am able to weigh this in one bowl.

Turn on the scale, it reads zero, toggle from ounces to grams, and set the bowl of beef stroganoff on top. Mine reads 8002g, minus 762g for the bowl, 8002-762=7240g, so my batch is 7240 grams, divided by 16, 7240÷16=452.5g or 452 grams per serving.

This meal is a pound of food! (for only 500 calories)

Ladies, you could likely eat half of this meal, and then the other half three hours from now, 250cal and 250cal, making this meal stretch 5-6 hours.

06:00 up
07:00 half Beef Stroganoff
10:00 half Beef Stroganoff
12:00 Lunch (say, NCD Chicken Caesar Salad)

Men, you're gonna love eating all this food. This meal is ten XLarge mouthfuls of food, mmm!

So weigh the batch, subtract the weight of the bowl, divide by 16, and aliquot it (divide it up) into 16 medium pyrex bowls. Place the pyrex bowl on the scale, turn on the scale, it will read zero, add beef stroganoff until it says 452 grams, cover with the red lid, repeat 15 more times, refrigerate them all.

Last step, the parsley.
Fill a large bowl with hot water, hold the parsley by the stems and submerge-and-up (dip wash) the parsley 6 times, flick it to remove water, then place it on a cutting board and chop off the stems, then chop it up, slicing it from one end to the other, then running your

knife over it back and forth a few times. Transfer the chopped parsley to a large pyrex bowl, cover and refrigerate it.

Tip. If your parsley is slightly wilted, place it in a plastic bag, add 1oz of water, tie a knot at the open end of the plastic bag to seal it, and toss it in the fridge. The next morning the parsley will be perky and firm.

Okay, that's it. The beef stroganoff is done and aliquoted into bowls, the parsley is grab-&-go ready, and the breadsticks we made earlier. Let's Eat!

Chapter 5

Let's Eat!

You can eat this from the bowl at your job, or serve it on a plate and eat at the table. This meal is fancy enough to serve to guests. And they will thank you for not overstuffing them with calories. Your guest will be able to go out to the backyard and play with the dog or swim in the pool, as the post-meal feel will make them feel like doing something, rather than sitting.

When I make this, it's still warm-hot when I have the first meal, so I place a plate on the scale, zero it, add 452g of beef stroganoff, remove the plate, take two breadsticks and break them into pieces on top of the beef stroganoff, then place the plate on the scale again, zero it (press tare), then add 10 grams of chopped parsley.

Mmmm!

Delicious.

The remaining meals I usually eat cold, but if I want it hot, add the two breadsticks to the bowl of beef stroganoff, cover with a paper towel, place it in the microwave and press 2:15, (this is hot, but not too hot), top with 10g of parsley, and sit down and eat. Mmm.

Heating it brings out the beef stroganoff flavor more.

Alternatively, you can omit the parsley, and heat it, and then it really has a lot of beef stroganoff flavor. Or, have every 4th meal with no parsley, so, meals 4 8 12 16 will be very beef stroganoff-y.

On the flipside, if you're like me, and my mom, then you enjoy the taste of the parsley mixed in, and so I often double or triple the parsley. In fact, I sometimes take a whole handful of parsley and put it on top, to make like a Beef Stroganoff Parsley salad! Mmm.

The parsley is not there to add color, it's there because it has flavor and contrast. Plus it's bright green and your body will say, "parsley parsley, I need parsley". Let your internals speak to you, rather than your eyes and mouth. Listen to your internals. The inner you.

Our final numbers are:
E=522
F=149
SF=81
TF=0
Chol=158
Na=355 (low in sodium)
CHO=214
nCHO=199
f=15
s=24 (very low in sugar) (5% sugar, 24/507x100)
Prot=144
T=507
42 29 28 (42+29+28=99% because it's rounding down)
T-f=492
With the T-f and nCHO it's 40.4 30.3 29.3 or basically 40 30 30.

The mushrooms have 16 calories of protein, and we didn't count them, so there's a bit more protein than 144. Bottom line, it's perfect as is, nutrition, numbers, and taste (fun).

Cost is $3.00 per meal.

Don't forget to tip the waiter on the way out! (that's you)
And give yourself a pat on the back for eating healthy.

Follow-up

1. If you eat caffeine, you feel jittery. If you eat 100% sugar, you feel hyper. If you eat 40 30 30, you feel Pumped Up! This meal is anabolic, aka, testosterone (youth hormone).

2. DO NOT overcook any of it, especially not the beef, or the noodles, because it you do, the flavor will not be the same. Overcooked beef tastes dead. The mushrooms need to be alive still. Set your timer and take notes. Write them into this book.

3. Coral Calcium is a great way to supplement with all the minerals, including those rare trace minerals. Open one capsule and sprinkle it on top, you won't even notice it.

4. If you made the NCD Blue Bran Muffins, then you had 176g of whipped butter left over. Use some of this leftover whipped butter in this recipe, but use 35 grams instead of 38. But if you use 38g of the whipped butter, it's not a big deal, only an extra 1.5 calories of fat per meal.

5. You will need a large restaurant-sized spatula to mix this bowl of beef stroganoff. I got mine at Smart & Final. To mix it, turn the bowl clockwise with your left hand, while mix-and-folding it over with the spatula in your right hand. Do this about 20 times.

6. This is not a boring or hard-to-eat meal. For example, I ate 2 meals the first day, then 4 the next day, then 4 the following day, and 4 the day after that, then 2, so 2 4 4 4 2 = 16 meals in 5 days. Or have it for breakfast and dinner for 8 days. It lasts 10 days.

7. Ten grams of chopped parsley is about $1/4^{th}$ of a cup, so double would be half a cup, and the handful for the salad version would be about a cup of parsley. Mmm. It's delicious! Try it.

8. If you are working out, your body will love this meal, it really is a meal that goes straight to your muscles and pumps you up. No matter what age you are, strength helps keep you young.

Leave a Review

If you are going to leave a review, first ask yourself:

1. Did the recipe target 40 30 30 and 500 calories? Yes it did.
2. Does the photo accurately depict the meal? Yes is does.
3. Was full disclosure made before you purchased? Yes it was.
   "With a side of entertainment!"
   (and if you're not a fan, just quietly move on, you don't need to
   spoil it for others and turn people away by being negative)

www.amazon.com   Search: NCD Beef Stroganoff

Subscribe to my YouTube Channel
www.youtube.com   ABC Water and the Number Crunch Diet

abcwaterandthenumbercrunchdiet@mail.com
Privacy – your email address will not be used for anything other
than by Jumper Publications and Media.
www.abcwaterandthenumbercrunchdiet.com

Some of you may have caught on that I'm using a different name.
Actually, those are my names, just in a different order. Amazon
allows authors to have up to three bio pages, but they have to be
different names, so I am able to double my exposure on their
website by using a different name. It's similar to how Safeway,
SuperValu, Vons, and Alberstons are all owned by Alberstons LLC.

Party On Dude

For those of you that want to read *ABC Water and the Number
Crunch Diet*, but it's a bit expensive for you, if you send me a
money order or PayPal payment I can mail you the book for 40%
off the list price ($108) and free shipping.

Learn everything you need to know about alkalinity and acid-base.

NUMBER CRUNCH DIET

01	Rueben Sandwich
02	Soyaki Chicken
03	Blue Bran Muffins
04	Beef Stroganoff
05a	Corn on the Cob
05b	Cola Milkshake
06a	Beef Jerky Cookies
06b	Peanut Butter Chocolate
07a	Steak Baked Beans
07b	Raw-Egg Eggnog
08	Chicken Caesar Salad
09a	Beef & Rice
09b	Orange Juice Milk – ADM
09c	Melted Cheddar – ADM
10	Chicken Potato Salad
11a	Beef Dip
11b	2% Milk Perfected
12	check back later
13	to follow
14	pending
15	to be published soon
16	not available yet
17	coming soon
18	not yet available
19	to be released in the fall
20	oops, error 404
21	please try again
22	it's been a busy week (month)(year!)
23	I'm workin' on it
24	coming to a theater near you
25	check again later

NUMBER CRUNCH DIET

26	pending
27	please check again later
28	system maintenance
29	check back later
30	later dude
31	refresh
32	not responding
33	crash dump
34	reboot
35	please wait
36	please be patient
37	loading…
38	page not available
39	check back later
40	please try again later
41	laters
42	partial
43	in process
44	processing
45	please check back
46	future release date pending
47	not yet available
48	my guess is
49	you will
50	Check Back Later ;)

Build a NCD Recipe Repertoire

Body –> Mind –> Soul => Spirit